Ileostomy

Top Twelve

Tips

For

Healthy Living

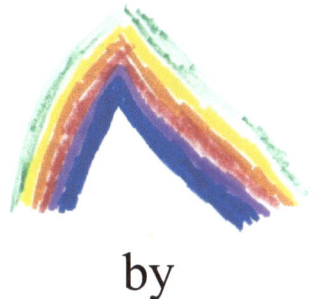

by

Louisa Paylor

Simple tips

to help you

live in harmony

with your

ostomy

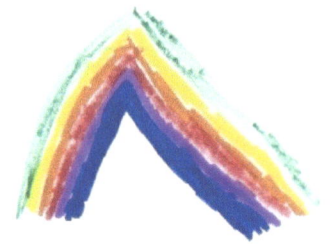

Ileostomy Top Twelve Tips for Healthy Living

by Louisa Paylor

First issue September 2017

ISBN: 9781549946851

Series: Healthy Living.

Book One

For my Mum

Who cared for me and my son thought out my illness and surgery

Who wholly supported me every step of the way.

Thank you, Mum.

For my Son

who has always been very encouraging

and

drew the rainbow for this guide.

Thank you, Son.

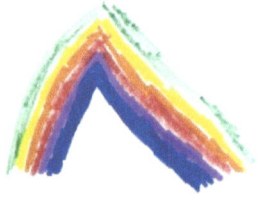

Introduction

I have written this guide to assist you in living with your ostomy; be it ileostomy, colostomy, stoma or indeed any other type of ostomy. An ostomy is where a small part of the large or small intestine is pulled out to assist with defecation with a bag attached over and around the ostomy as the large bowl (the colon) or the small intestine (ileum) are not working correctly. For the purpose of this guide I will use the term ostomy throughout.

There is a list of definitions for you at the back of this guide.

The journey to any ostomy is a bumpy one and is sometimes sprung on people who wake from surgery with no idea of what or how to manage life with an ostomy.

I was lucky enough to have the choice of an ileostomy or an internal 'J' pouch. I can happily say I choose 'Harry' (my ileostomy). I have lived with Harry for 6 years now as I write this for you in 2017.

As you read this, I want you to know I am with you. Now, let's start with what is your ostomy called?

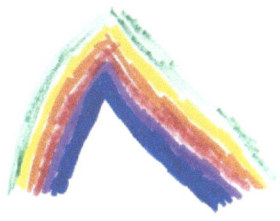

Top Tip One

Give your ostomy a name.

'I am sorting out Harry' I say to my family as I go to the bathroom. This is so they know I will be in the bathroom for a bit longer. It helps give them more patience with me. Or if out and about, I can refer to Harry instead the tongue twisting name ileostomy.

I was advised to do this at the hospital I had my surgery. It has proved to be good advice. To give an ostomy a name such as 'Harry' is to give it a 'he or she' element to make them personal.

I know others called Stanley and Humphrey.

I feel this is the important first tip. As half the battle of living well with your ostomy is a positive outlook.

"I accept my ostomy. I am thankful for him (or her)"

Top Tip Two

Always wash your hands with a good soap after every visit to the loo.

I have learnt from painful experience that hands can become sore and dry from frequent washing. I recommend using a very gentle moisturising soap.

I use Dove beauty cream bar soap every time I use the bathroom. This helps to keep my hands soft with less chance of painful cracked fingers around the nails which can happen if my skin becomes too dry.

Added to this, I would strongly recommend always using a good, moisture rich hand cream after washing. I like to use the Sanctuary Spa hand cream. Once a month I like to do the Champneys intensive overnight hand therapy which really helps to rejuvenate my hands and keep them silky smooth and healthy.

"My hands are soft and supple"

Top Tip Three

Deodorizing absorbent sachets.

These are available on NHS prescription.

Deodorizing absorbent sachets will make the poop solidify the liquid into a more poop like substance helping to remove the smell. They also help to make a leak a less dramatic event.

When a new bag is put over Harry I will add 2 sachets, pushing them into the body of the bag. They absorb the liquid and then the poop becomes a bit like lumpy poop or crystals depending on how many you use. After emptying the bag, I add two more sachets into the end of the bag opening. The sachets then do their deodorizing and absorbencies ready for the next loo visit where I repeat the process again.

You will leak, everyone does, and it's how you deal with it that counts. I have written about my first leak in the men's changing room in M&S at the back of this book.

"My bag always performs well for me"

Top Tip Four

Flanges.

These are available on NHS prescription.

These are sticky-back curved stripes that go around the edges of your bag slightly covering the flange edge on the bag attached to your body. This gives an extra layer of protection. They can be half or quarter in size. If half size, you will generally need two to go around the whole bag.

Flanges are good to keep with you if you are out and your bag starts to leak and you cannot change it straight away. These can be used to reinforce the bag until you can get home or to a place where you can change the bag.

If you are a little nervous of an outing you have not done with your ostomy before or you are out for the whole day. Add flanges around the edge of your bag. This gives you reassurance and confidence that your bag is secure and will not leak.

"I always have the best products available to me"

Top Tip Five

Salt.

I remember being told at the hospital that without a colon it is more difficult to absorb the salt from foods that I need as part of a healthy diet. I then read that to put a pinch of salt in 1 litre of made up squash per day creates an energy drink. My doctor approved of this. Taken with food this also aids digestive absorption.

A sewn up back-end can get sore and painful. Adding a handful or two of sea salt to a bath will help to relieve the soreness and inflammation. If I become really sore and uncomfortable, I use Sudocrem 'antiseptic healing cream'. I cannot think of another cream that does the job as well.

When I use sun cream or a moisturiser in the day and then wish to bathe before an evening out. I will shower rather than bath. This is because the oils in the sun cream and moisturisers can interfere with a new bag not sticking properly. A leak overnight after a lovely evening out is not acceptable to me!

"I am comfortable, safe and secure at all times"

Top **T i p S i x**

Keep essentials in your makeup bag.

I always keep absorbent gel sachets, flanges and a small handy pack of mini wipes in my makeup bag. The sachets I use every time I empty Harry's bag and the flanges are there if I happen to start a leak and it's not convenient to change him.

Mini wipes, I buy from the supermarket. I use them in the day when out at work or shopping to help clean the opening end of the bag once it is emptied before I add the gel sachets.

In time, you will learn your own essentials to keep by you.

"I am always well prepared for every outing"

Top Tip Seven

Get a disabled toilet key.

These cost about £3:00 from you local (UK) council. Anyone can request one without an interrogation!

The disabled toilets have a higher seat which makes emptying an ostomy bag a lot easier.

The facility is there for you to change or empty your bag in a private place, without having to wait for a regular loo.

Also I find some regular public toilets are just too small to move around in when dealing with Harry's bag.

"A toilet facility is available to me whenever I need one"

Top Tip Eight

Pants.

It is important to discuss with your Stoma Nurse where the site of your ostomy will be before surgery so you are comfortable with it. It is usually sited below the jeans belt line. This is, of course, the ideal scenario. Some are done in emergency operations but your excellent surgeon will site it well for you.

I find any 'Bridget Jones style' full brief pants are fine in general. These are available anywhere that sell pants. Full pants will let your ostomy bag sit snugly within them and the pants usually come up to your natural waist line. There are those of you would who like a smaller brief, do recommend them to us.

Cotton is best as I find a synthetic material can make me sweat and this can cause Harry's bag to become unstuck.

In the summer, I wear Comfizz pants. These are ostomy support pants. They are secure and give me confidence when I am wearing a summer dress. They can also give me a little tummy support if I eat too much cake!

Comfizz supply specialist support wear for ostomies:

pants, vest and belts of differing support levels.

They have a great website with bloggers, advice and inspirational stories from people living with their ostomy.

comfizz.com

Some of Comfizz products are available on the NHS prescription service. They also have a range for children.

"I am comfortable and confident wherever I am"

Top Tip Nine

Toilets.

Toilets come in all shapes and sizes, I recently worked in an office block where the all the toilet blocks were refurbished and replaced from industrial to modern domestic U-bend toilets, and it goes without saying that they soon put signs up saying no wipes down the loo! The same happened at my son's school.

The height of a loo will matter, when deciding whether you can empty your bag while sitting on the loo or you need to kneel to empty it. This is why the public disabled loos are great as they are extra large.

I regularly put bleach down the loo before I use it. That prevents much of the smell.

A couple of drops of Lavender oil in the cistern once a week gives your loo a lovely fragrance.

"My flush, I bless. I am thankful and grateful for the plumbing"

Top Tip Ten

Bags.

I can only go on my own experience for this one. There is a good choice of bags available and you really need to work with your stoma nurse for support.

I use two types of bags. Dansac Novalife Midi is a smaller drainable bag, which as a swimmer, once wet still holds it stick well. I have even been known to leave it on for a day or two, especially on holiday.

For those moments when I eat too much mashed potato and the poop works its way under the edge of the bag and creates soreness because of the acid in the poop. (I think this is known as pancaking) I use Salts Confidence Be drainable. Which is larger and is award winning having researched into 'healthy stoma skin'. And comes in a variety of colours.

"I always make the right choices for me"

Top Tip Eleven

Join a Support Group.

A good group will have talks and demonstrations from representatives of different organisations that provide products and services to ostomy users. You could also sample or trial new products. There will be outings, pub and dinner events. You can learn a lot from each other.

Look around your local area and ask your stoma nurse who will have details of local groups. If not, start your own.

IA, the ileostomy & internal pouch support group has a list of local groups you can join and a helpful website with lots of useful information on living with an ostomy. www.iasupport.org

Colostomy UK (formerly the colostomy association) has a website packed full of useful information on every aspect of ostomy life and care. They have a list of stoma support groups and even offer advice on how you can start a group. www.colostomyuk.org

"I am surrounded by people who appreciate me"

Top Tip Twelve

Donate you unused bags and flanges.

Here in the UK we are blessed to have many of our ostomy products available through the NHS or at subsidised costs for us.

There are many in the developing world that do not have access to ostomy products and use crisp packets, tin cans or plastic bags to put around the ostomy, secured with string or elastic bands. This has a high risk of infection. It must be stressful and can be very isolating for the person.

Stoma Aid project is a charity which will take all your unwanted bags and flanges and organises them to be sent to developing countries. The colostomy website has a page with further information. Or you can send your unused bags and flanges (only) to this address:

Stoma Aid
c/o Stone Logistics/PRS Ltd
Lorne Mill
Lorne Street
Bolton
BL4 7LZ

I am happy, health and contented

I have vibrant health and energy

I accept parts of my body I cannot change

I respect my body's changing needs and desires

I am thankful and grateful for Harry"

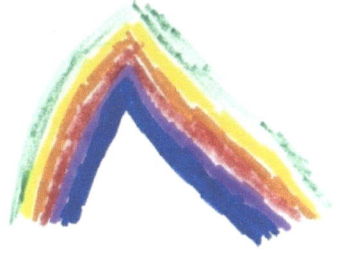

Medical names and terms

Ileostomy - a part of the small intestine, ileum is used to create an external opening for bowel movements to be excreted on the right side of the body.

Colostomy - a part of the colon is used to externally create an opening for bowel movements to be excreted from on the left side of the body.

Ostomy - term given to anyone with either an ileostomy or colostomy.

Stoma – commonly used with reference to a colostomy

Stoma nurse – (titles may change in time) who commonly assist with all ostomy support from surgery to everyday care.

Defecation – a posh word for pooing.

Flanges – the edge of the ostomy bag that sticks to your body. Also the name of the sticky strips you can add to your bag for extra security.

Rested – a term given between operations to give the body time to recover before the next surgery is needed. An ostomy will generally need two or three operations to complete the final procedure.

Internal Pouch/J Pouch – a new reservoir is surgically created where the bowel and anus have been removed to store bowel contents for passing as poop.

Mesalazine – an inflammatory resistant drug commonly used in the treatments for ulcerative colitis.

Cyclosporine – an immune-suppressant medication used to treat acute sever ulcerative colitis usually given by intravenous drip direct into a vein.

Arsenic - suppositories (Aceartol) used to treat ulcerative colitis.

Suppositories – a bullet shaped tablet that is inserted into the rectum to allow a quick, direct absorbency of the drug.

My Story

My son was born in 2007, a joy from a very difficult and stressful relationship. I soon became a single devoted Mum. Then in 2008 I was diagnosed with ulcerative colitis; following on from this were two years of difficult treatment as I was intolerant to the key ingredient of most of the treatments of colitis: Mesalazine. This involved some long stays in hospital and with a young baby this was not acceptable to me. I was soon transferred from Watford General Hospital to St Marks Hospital the specialist bowel hospital in Harrow, Middlesex.

It became clear that no medication could control the colitis so in 2011 most of my colon was removed with the remaining 10cm left for a new internal pouch to be made.

I was rested (a term given to the period between operations) with Harry (the name I gave my ileostomy) for 5 months. I was happy to be free from hospital visits and home with my young son. I was able to take him to school. We went on holiday; swam and biked. I was living again. I was happy and contemplating keeping Harry.

I was due to have the second operation in June to build the new internal pouch using the last 10 cm of my colon remaining for this procedure. Unfortunately the last 10 cm of colon flared. This time steroids did not work. Due to my intolerance to Mesalazine my options were limited. My consultants wanted to admit me to hospital for Cyclosporine by intravenous drip. I said no as I did not want to leave my son again. The consultants discussed this and came back to say they did not usually do this but they could put me on arsenic suppositories (Aceartol) for a short time. This worked and my second operation was booked for October.

I now had time to think and research about whether to keep Harry or choose the option of an internal pouch. We were soon organising the school summer holidays. Then in July I had a call from the hospital saying as my bowel was calm they would like to do the second operation as soon as possible in August.

I was not ready for this. I was not convinced having an internal pouch was right for me as the last 10cm of colon had flared with colitis. To build a new internal pouch with this remaining colon would mean regular hospital visits with the possibility of further colitis flare ups and even possibly cancer in the remaining colon.

I thought I had to try the internal pouch for ease of lifestyle. My indecision went on right up to the morning of the op. The surgeon had phoned me to discuss this the day before. He said he did not mind which op he did, to remove the last 10cm with a permanent ileostomy or to make an internal pouch.

At the hospital on the morning of the surgery, the surgeon sent one of his doctors upstairs twice to ask me what I wanted to do. I had emailed St Marks specialist stoma nurse Zarah the day before and she came and talked with me. It was Zarah who made me realise I must trust my inner feelings and keep Harry and not go for the internal pouch. We agreed and she got my notes and wrote across the front in black ink 'no pouch' for the surgeon. She went and told him personally as well. I walked to the theatre waving to my mum happy, knowing I had made the right choice and a new awareness to trust my inner guide more.

I have given thanks to my mum at the beginning of this book. I really feel I need to say thank you again here as mum is the 'we' in this story. She lost her husband to cancer when I was ill with colitis and though grieving, mum looked after her grandson. She came to visit me in hospital with clean pj's and stocks of essentials and would be home in time to collect him from nursery. She really was his main carer for three years and a great help to me with all the household chores and without her I would not have managed my illness and my son. I hope that one day she will write her story from a carer's point of view, as they are the unsung heroes in many cases.

I have had Harry for 6 years now. I am thankful and grateful I tell him this every day. I say sorry if I eat anything that he finds hard to dispel or if he has too much gas to deal with. 'I listen to and follow my body's needs and desires'.

I realise now that my colitis was an emotional response to do with not letting go, holding on to old destructive negative thoughts and feelings of the difficult relationship with my son's father. It is a lesson I am continuing to learn.

In the last three years, I have had very personal issues to deal with. There was never going to be an apology or explanation for unacceptable behaviour. The anger, frustration and betrayal started to make me sick again. I prayed for guidance to help me let go of the situation. This came in the book 'Living Magically' by Gill Edwards. It helped me find the art of letting go in accepting, forgiveness and love. I went on to read more inspirational books. I discovered meditation through yoga and then found online guided meditations and videos. I came across Hay House which has been of great guidance and inspiration to me. I list my resources in the back of this guide for you.

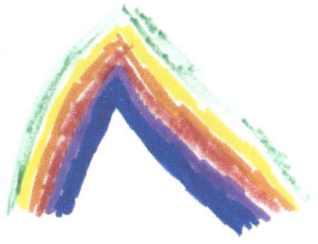

The first leak

In the early days, 1 was not experienced with Harry nor did I have a proper routine. One morning I showered and changed Harry's bag. It was summer and a hot day.

My partner (then) and I went to town shopping for some new trousers for him and we parked in the multi storey car park. I had got used to leaving a small makeup bag of Harry's supplies in the glove compartment of the car. It had been in my handbag, but I had never used it so left it in the car.

We went into a few shops when I started to feel that Harry's bag was uncomfortable. We were in M & S men's changing rooms for my partner to try on trousers. I felt an uncomfortable feeling I know so well now of the burning poop working its way under the flange of the bags edge but I didn't then. I asked him if he could just step outside the door while I checked Harry. I put my hand down and a felt squidgy poop and noticed a smell. This was before I used absorbent sachets. He said he could smell it too! I had to change Harry but the bag was in the car. I was in a high state of anxiety and emotion.

At this point, my partner left me and when into town. I was left to get upstairs to the car park, four floors up and get the bag and then get down to the M & S disabled loo.

By this time I was in a real mess and poop, bag and pants went in the bin, Harry was really active and doing his wonderful job of spewing out poop. I ran out of wipes. Someone banged on the door. The bag I had put on would not stick I was shaking so much. I tried another, now panicking I was in the disabled loo and someone more deserving needed it. Would I be told off when I got out? The second bag stuck and I cleaned the loo, sink and floor!

I pulled myself together to have the courage to open the door. I was still in a very emotional state. I took a deep breath and opened the door. A security guard was standing there with about 6 people waiting for the toilets all staring at me. He rushed straight into the loo I had been in. My first thought was that he was checking for drugs! I felt like a criminal. Guilty and ashamed for taking what felt like 3 hours but was probably ½ hour, I walked out into the men's department and sat on one of the display stands and wept. I felt so alone and embarrassed.

I phoned my partner and could get no answer. I just wanted to go home. I really did not feel like walking to the high street to find him. But I had no choice. I found him half way up the high street. He said he left me as he did not know how to handle the situation. He could not understand why I was crying. We went home then.

I have to say that was 5 years ago. We parted ways going on to our own life paths. I have since had a lovely holiday romance with a wonderful chap who does not worry about Harry's pooping sounds, smells or the need for any special pants to 'aid' during making love. He loves me as I am and accepts Harry as a part of me.

Conclusion

I wanted to tell you this as it was my first public leak. There have been others, thought never as bad as that one was emotionally.

I am now in a more positive place and accept that leaks happen. I can often tell when it will occur if I make the hole too big or eat at the wrong time of day for me or have to many nuts or mash potato!

If Harry is spewing poop out into the bag and it needs to be pushed down, this cannot be done very well in a public place. I have had to sit through meetings knowing I will have to change Harry at the first available moment. As I have not been able to release the poop into the bag as it pushes its way out under the flange edge. People in my meetings have no idea what's going on in my pants! I just carry on as normal. To know all these things comes with time and experience.

Accepting that sometimes these things happen is part of having an ostomy and knowing he or she is doing a wonderful job to keep you alive and healthy. Love and accept that he or she is a

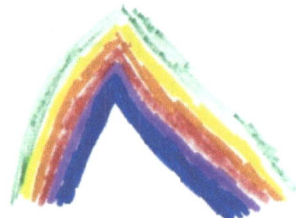

part of you and bless them.

Thank You

I would like to thank Zarah: St Marks Hospital specialist stoma nurse.

Carla and Nic my first ostomates to read it and tell me it was funny and useful to them. Gary and Andy for editorial help.

Rebecca whose help and assistance has been professional and priceless. Tracy thank you for being you and introducing me to IFS.

For the life that was Gill Edwards who started me of on this new path of my magical life.

Hay House for their guidance with weekly and monthly newsletters, online tutorials, videos and books.

Books

These are the books I have read that have helped to change the course of my life:

The Charkas - Hilary H Carter

Living Magically – Gill Edwards

Heal Your Life and Heal Your Body - Louise Hay

Goddesses Never Age - Dr Christiane Northrup

The Power of Now – Eckhart Tolle

Apologies:

To the men, I have no experience of a male ostomy. I am calling on you to write one!

Do get in touch

I hope you have found this useful, whether you are new to your ostomy or equally if you have had one for years and are learning a new way to view your ostomy.

I would love to hear your comments and suggestions.

Email me at: helloileolove@gmail.com

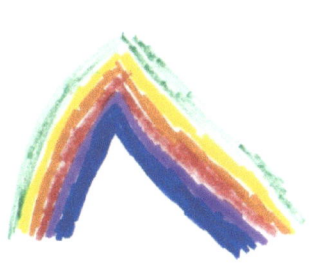